Spunky the Monkey

An Adventure In Exercise

WRITTEN BY LEN SAUNDERS

ILLUSTRATED BY DALE MOORE

AuthorHouse™
1663 Liberty Drive
Bloomington, IN 47403
www.authorhouse.com
Phone: 1-800-839-8640

First published by AuthorHouse 1/25/2010

ISBN: 978-1-4389-3991-9 (sc)

Printed in the United States of America
Bloomington, Indiana

This book is printed on acid-free paper.

For additional copies of this publication, please visit: www.lensaunders.com/books

authorHOUSE®

Dedicated with love to

Julie, Evan, and Ryan

A Message From Spunky

Dear Children:

I hope you enjoy my exercise adventure through the forest. Please read this book and exercise along with it every day. Each page will explain my special journey, as well as give you a suggestion on how to make the same movements I make through the forest. Use the daily checklist in the back of the book to keep track of your success. It is always important to stop exercising if you get very tired or you hurt yourself. Make sure an adult is in the room when you are exercising, and be sure you perform exercises that are considered safe for you. Have fun.

Love,
Spunky

Dear Parents And Teachers:

Please visit my Web site to see demonstrations of each exercise. Your children will love to exercise along with the images on the Web site for some healthy fun.

http://www.lensaunders.com/spunky

Love,

Spunky

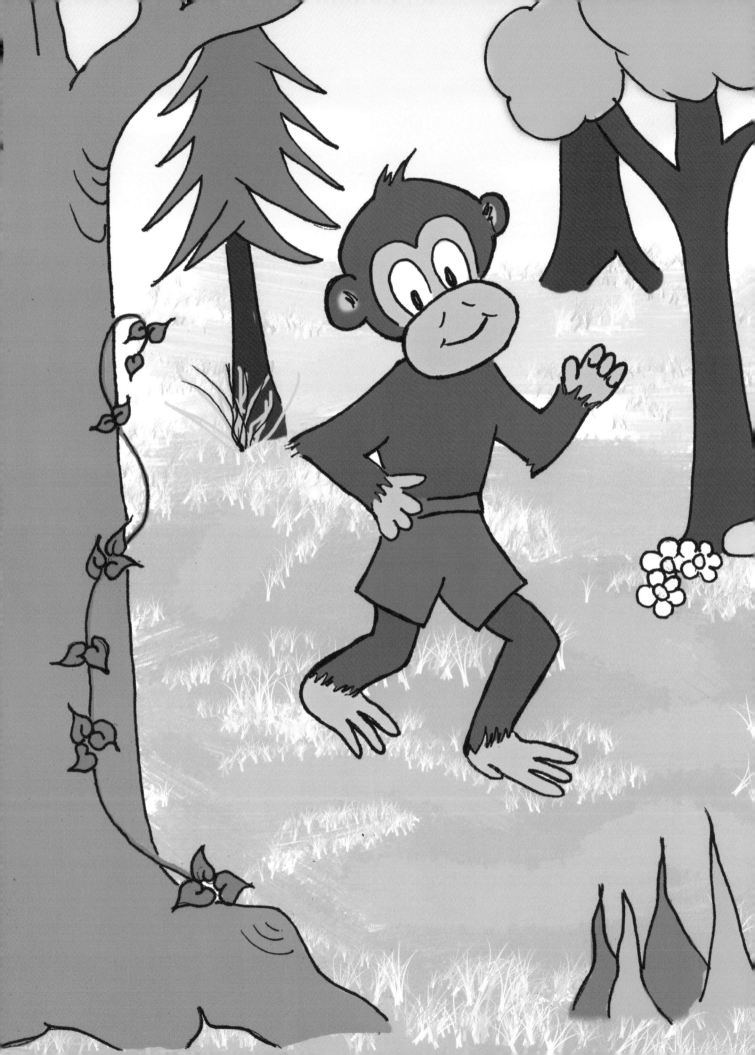

Spunky the Monkey loves
to run and play,
his adventure through the
forest began a great day.

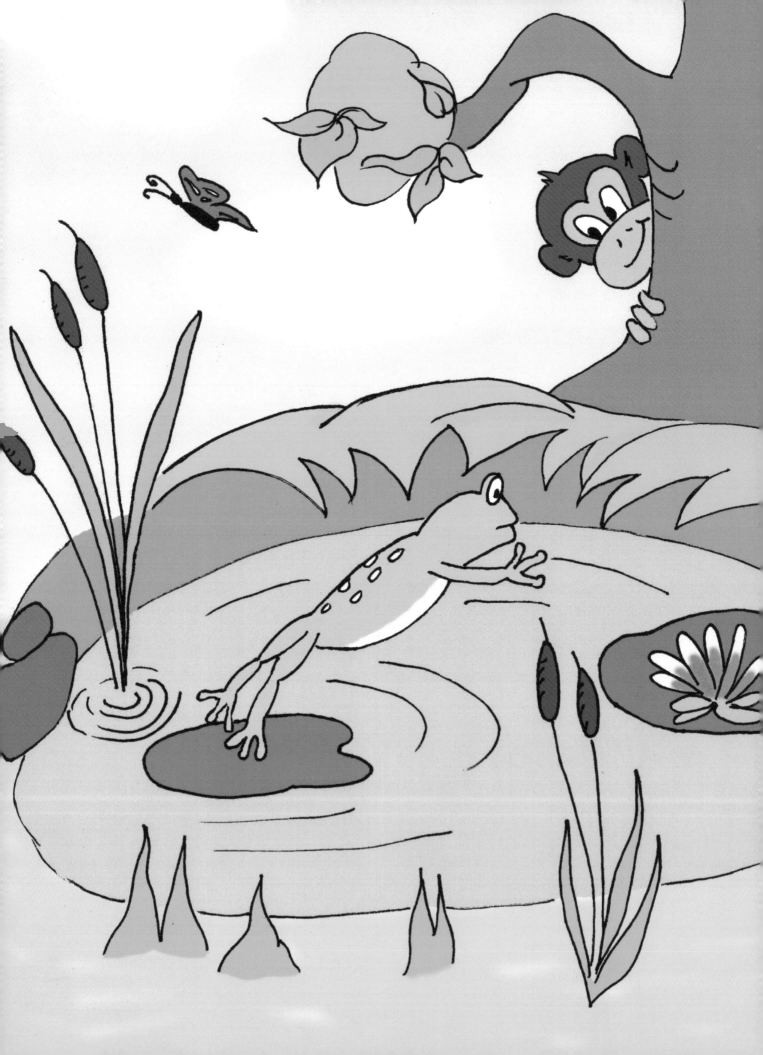

Spunky watched a frog jump from lily to lily, spinning and jumping and acting really silly.

Suggestion Box:

Can you imagine that you are a frog jumping and spinning from one lily pad to another lily pad? At home, imagine you have lily pads all over the floor. Carefully, start to jump from one imaginary lily pad to the next. Try to keep jumping for one minute.

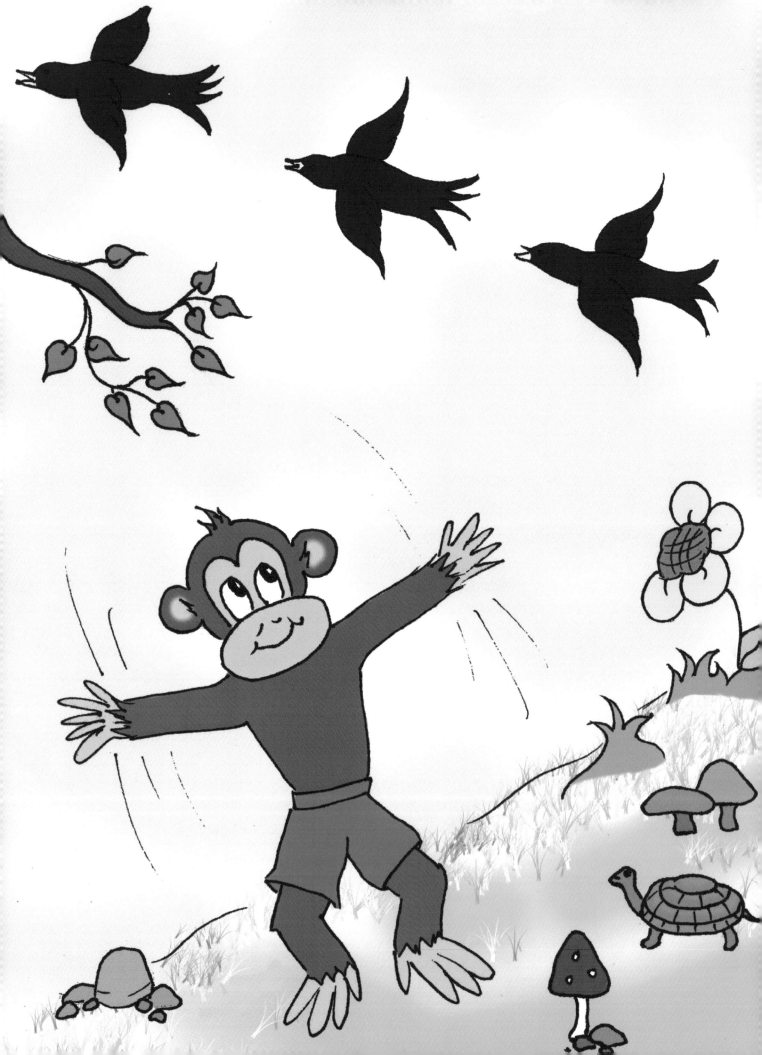

Spunky saw several birds flying up in the sky,

flapping their wings and soaring so high.

Suggestion Box:

Can you imagine you are a bird flying? Try moving your arms up and down twenty times like you are flapping your wings. Now try running around the room while you move your arms up and down for one minute.

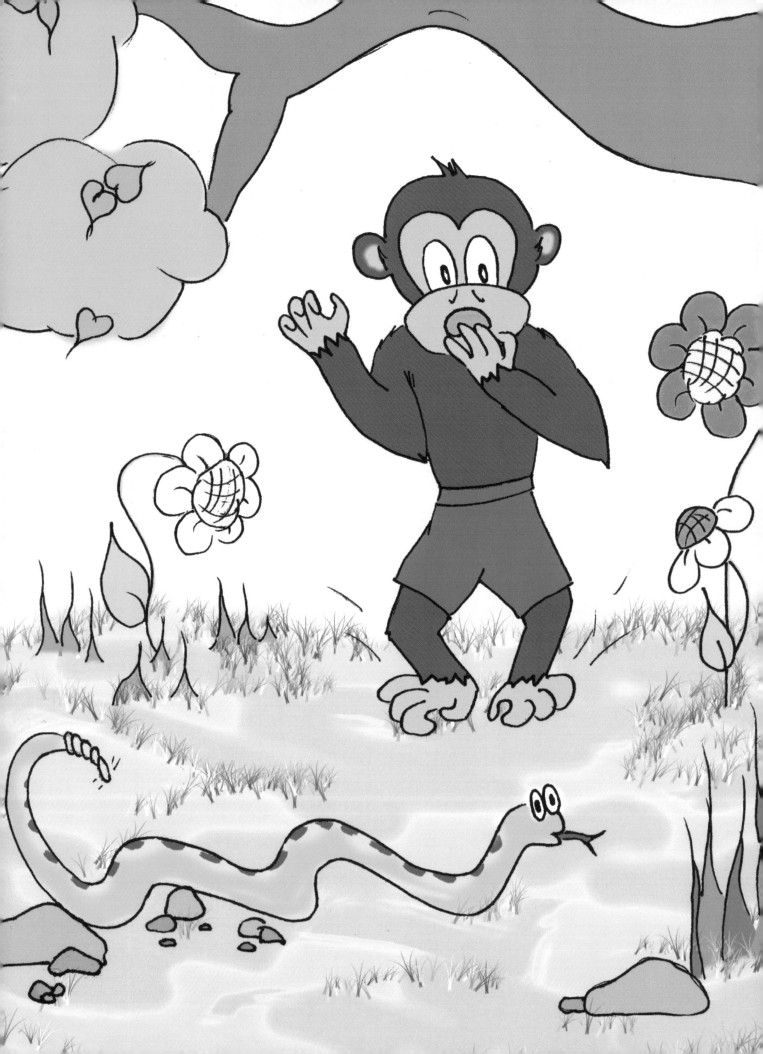

Spunky was startled when he heard a rattle and shake; slithering on the forest floor was a giant green snake.

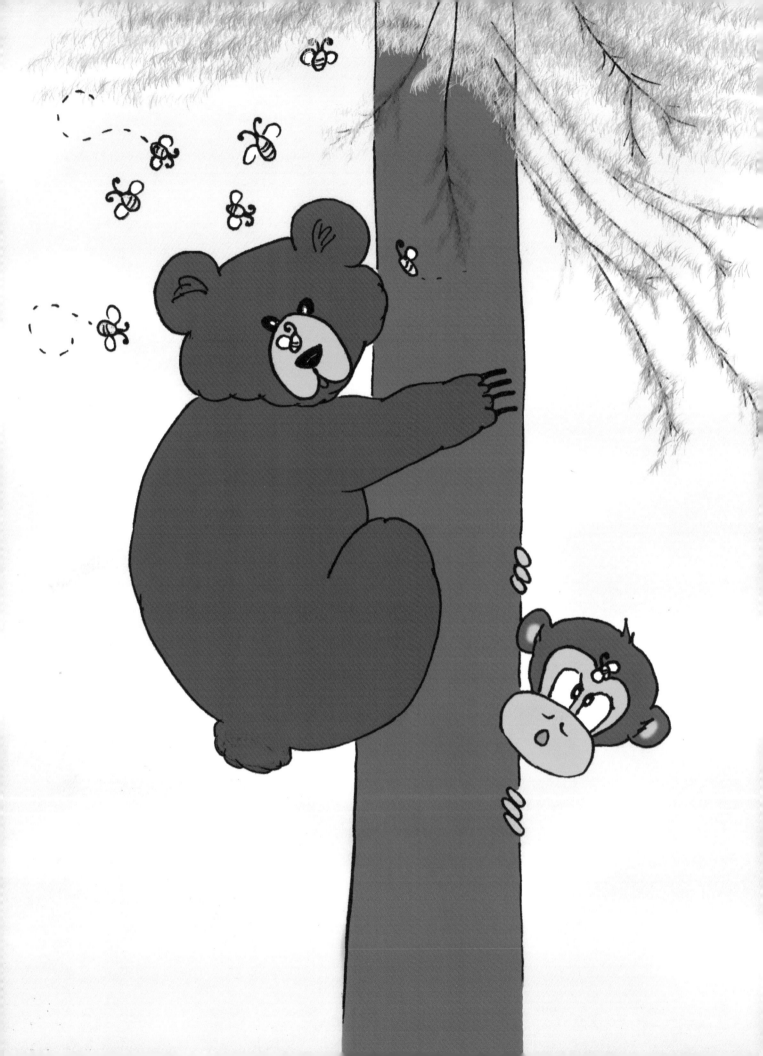

Spunky heard a loud
growl from the top of the
trees;
it was a bear eating honey
surrounded by bees.

Suggestion Box:

Can you imagine that you are a bear climbing a tree? Put
your hands above your head and move your arms up and
down while your legs walk in place. Did you make it to
the top of the tree?

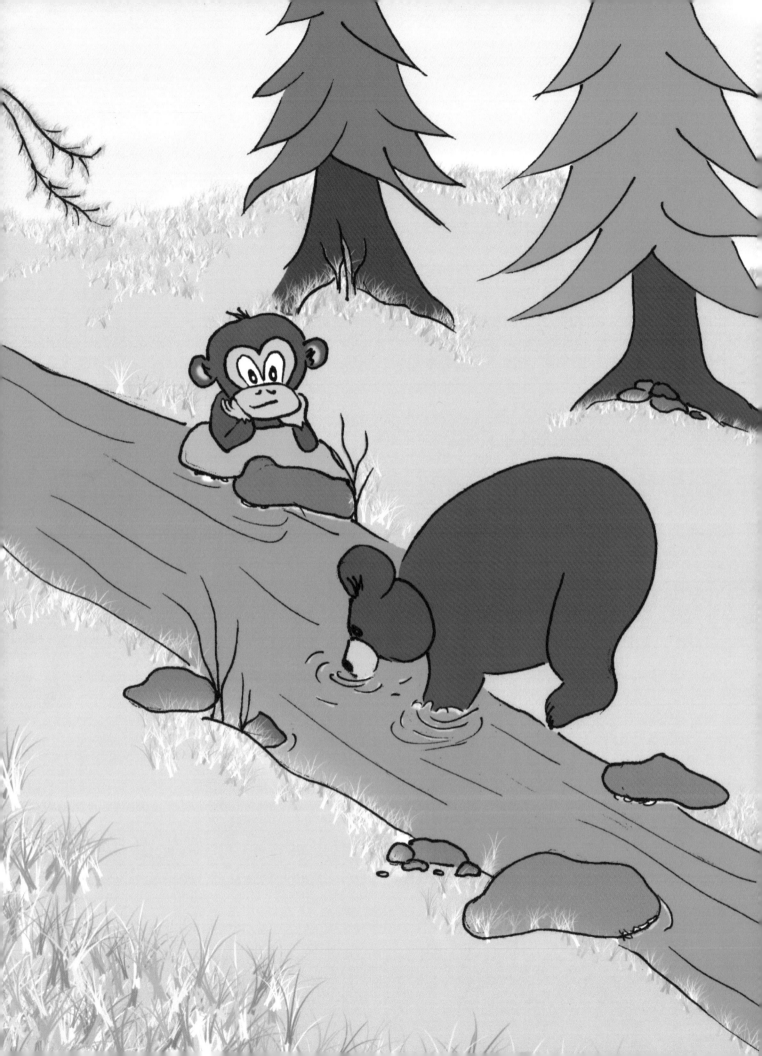

A cub was drinking water at the edge of a creek, moving up and down between each sip and peek.

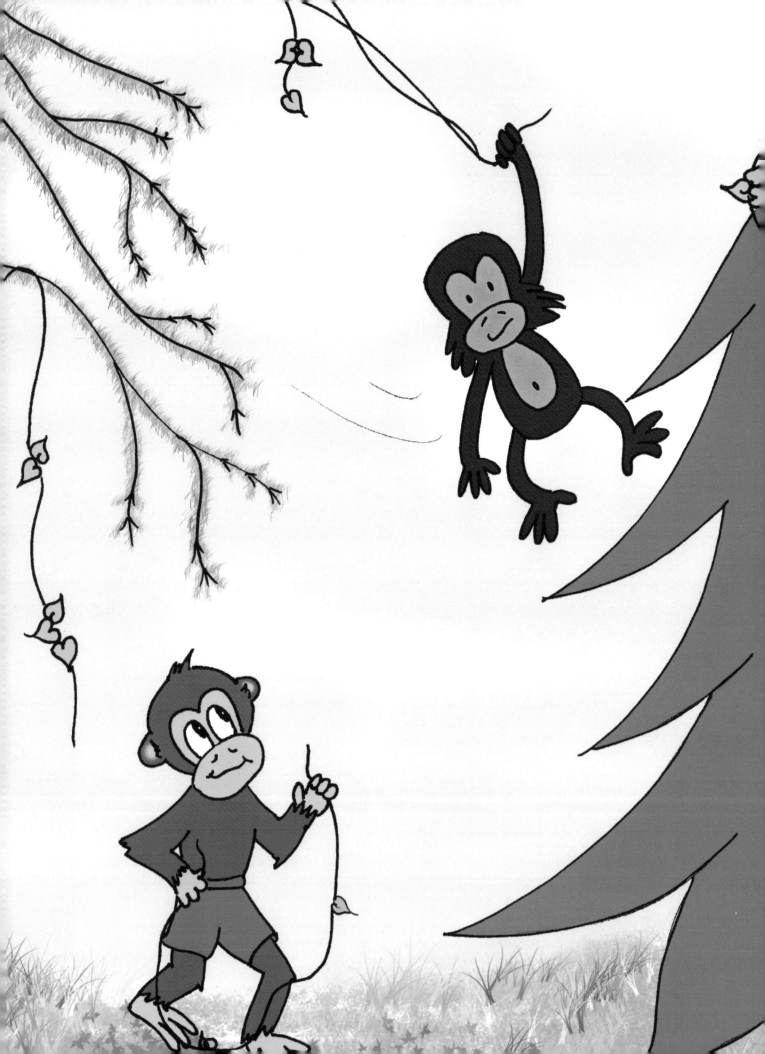

Spunky saw a small
chimp swinging high in
the vines;
she appeared to be
jumping rope between the
two pines.

Suggestion Box:

Can you imagine you are jumping rope? Leap in the air
and move your arms like you are jumping rope for ten
seconds. If that is too easy, try using a real jump rope.
Can you jump rope twenty times?

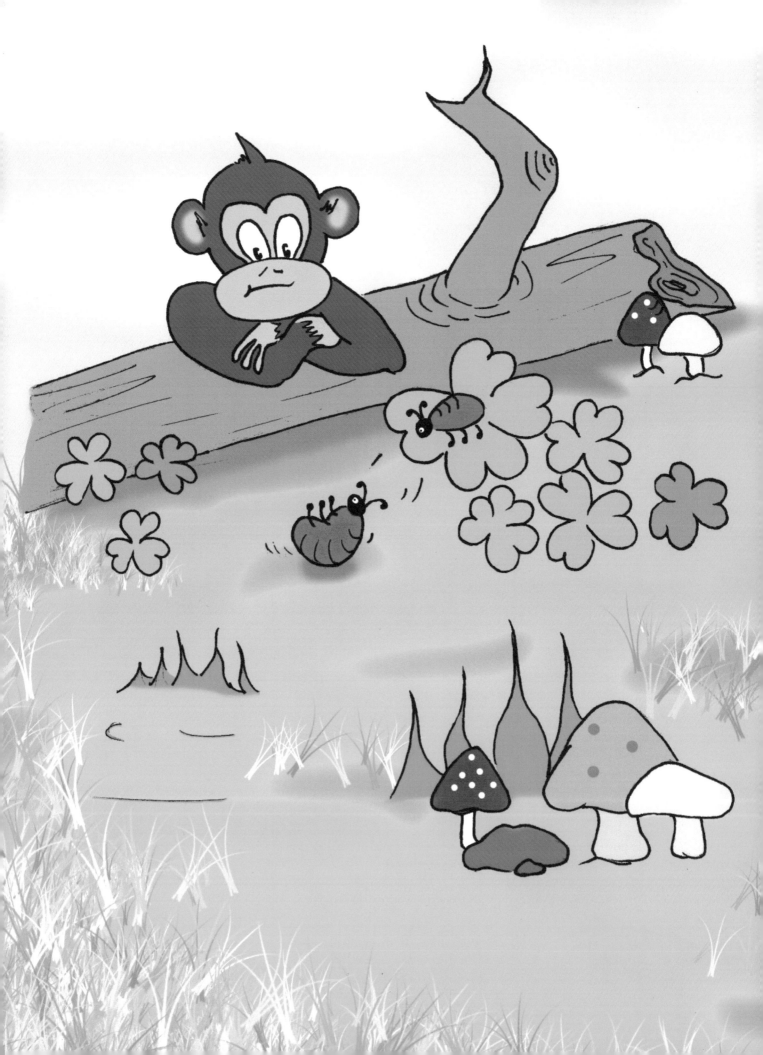

Spunky watched a beetle
fall from a clover;

he was trying to sit up and
flip back over.

Suggestion Box:

Can you think of an exercise that looks like a beetle
trying to sit up? How about a curl-up? Can you do five
curl-ups? Have a grown up hold your feet
while you try it.

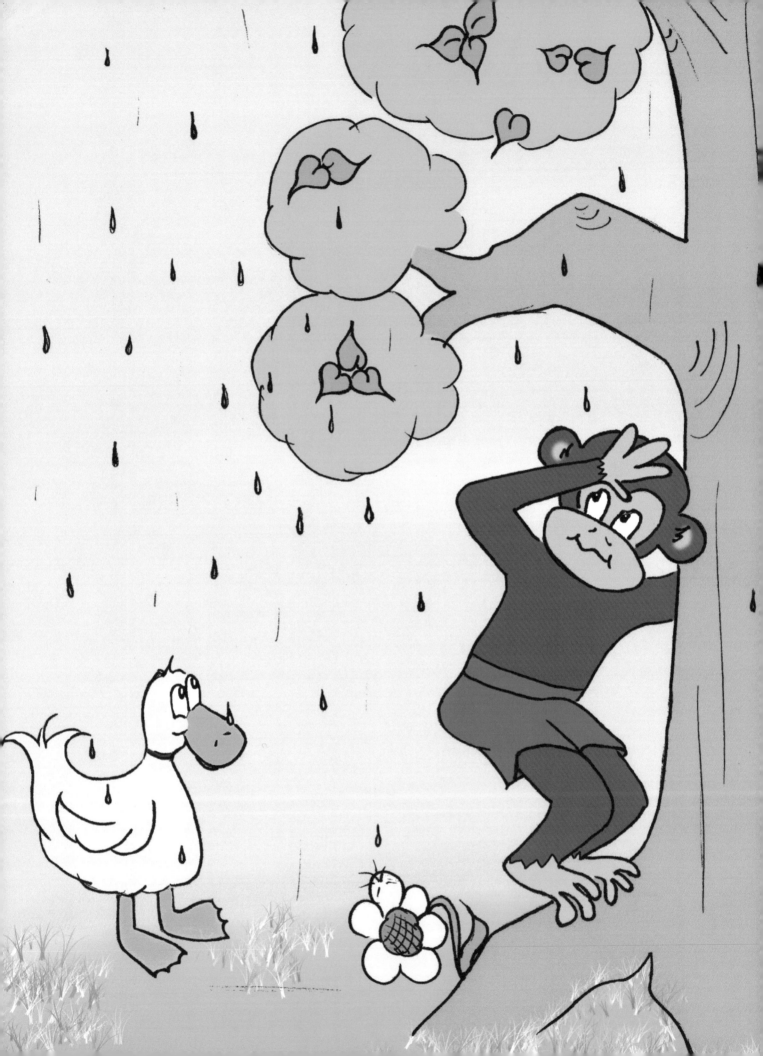

As the clouds started to thicken and rain fell from the sky,

Spunky jumped left and then right, trying to keep dry.

Suggestion Box:

Can you imagine rain falling on your head right now? Try not to get wet. Jump left, jump right, jump backward, and then quickly jump forward so the raindrops do not get you wet. Can you do that pattern two times?

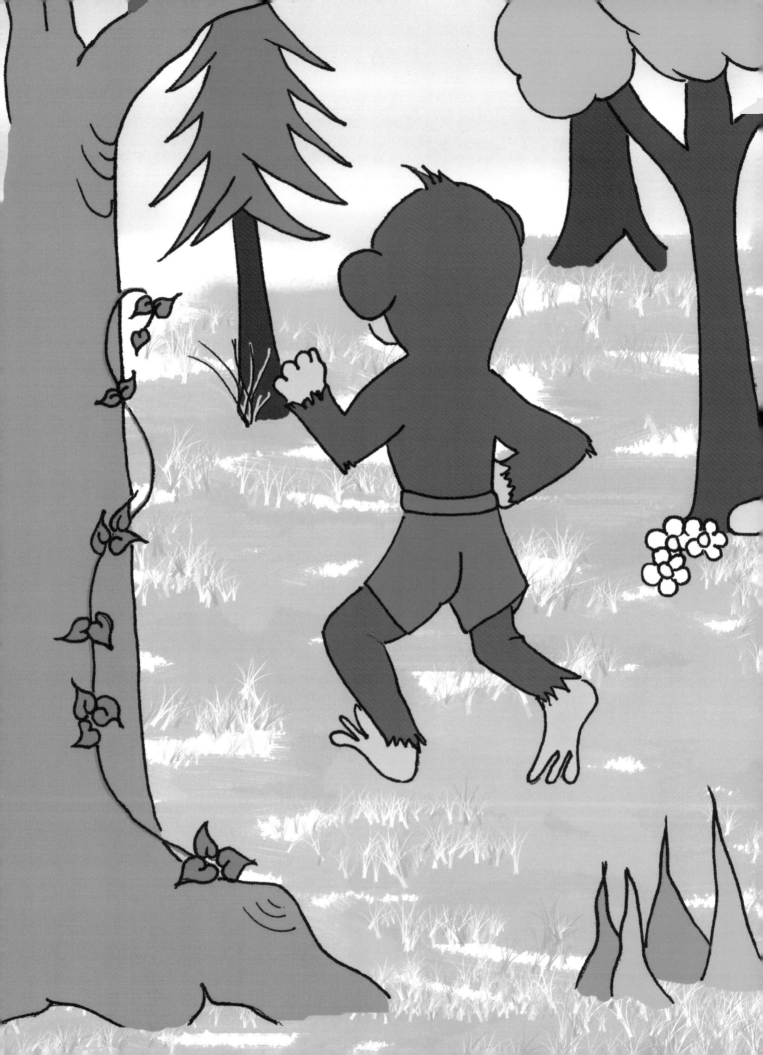

The sun came back out, and Spunky's adventure was through;

the main lesson he learned: exercise is good for you.

Suggestion Box:

What was your favorite exercise from this book? Try it again with a parent.

Monday

Run in Place:

Level 1: Have your child run in place for twenty seconds, rest, and then do it again.

Level 2: Have your child run in place for forty seconds.

Level 3: Have your child run in place for sixty seconds while simultaneously clapping his or her hands.

Spin and Jump:

Level 1: Have your child try to jump and spin from one imaginary lily pad to another lily pad on the floor.

Level 2: Have your child jump back and forth five times between two imaginary lily pads on the floor.

Level 3: Have your child jump back and forth between two imaginary lily pads on the floor for two minutes.

Fill in the blanks below every day when your child completes an exercise. Give him or her a star as you record participation. Examples are given below.

Run in Place Exercise Checklist

Sunday	Monday	Tuesday	Wednesday	Thursday	Friday	Saturday
	★ 60 seconds					

Spin and Jump Exercise Checklist

Sunday	Monday	Tuesday	Wednesday	Thursday	Friday	Saturday
	★ 2 minutes					

Tuesday

Arm Lifts:

Level 1: Have your child do twenty arm lifts in place as if he or she is flapping a pair of wings.

Level 2: Have your child perform a slow jog around the room while flapping his or her arms up and down twenty times.

Level 3: Have your child perform a slow jog around the room while flapping his or her arms up and down for two minutes.

Slithering:

Level 1: Have your child slither like a snake from one wall to another.

Level 2: Have your child slither from one wall to another two times at a faster pace.

Level 3: Have your child slither at a fast pace for one minute.

Fill in the blanks below every day when your child completes an exercise. Give him or her a star as you record participation. Examples are given below.

Arm Lifts Exercise Checklist

Sunday	Monday	Tuesday	Wednesday	Thursday	Friday	Saturday
		★ 35 arm lifts				

Slithering Exercise Checklist

Sunday	Monday	Tuesday	Wednesday	Thursday	Friday	Saturday
		★ 1 minute				

Wednesday

Step and climb:

Level 1: Have your child try walking in place while moving his or her arms as if climbing a tree for twenty seconds.

Level 2: Have your child try walking in place while moving his or her arms as if climbing a tree for forty seconds.

Level 3: Have your child try walking in place while moving his or her arms as if climbing a tree for sixty seconds.

Push-up:

Level 1: Have your child simulate bending up and down like he or she is drinking water from a pond. Then have him ore her try five push-ups.

Level 2: Have your child try ten push-ups.

Level 3: Have your child try twenty push-ups.

Fill in the blanks below every day when your child completes an exercise. Give him or her a star as you record participation. Examples are given below.

Step and Climb Exercise Checklist

Sunday	Monday	Tuesday	Wednesday	Thursday	Friday	Saturday
			★ 40 seconds			

Push-up Exercise Checklist

Sunday	Monday	Tuesday	Wednesday	Thursday	Friday	Saturday
			★ 5 push-ups			